www.anykindapills.com

START YOUR NEW HEALTHY LIFE NOW!

By Franck Bale

Copyright © 2014

Disclaimer

All the material contained in this book is provided for educational and informational purposes only. No responsibility can be taken for any results or outcomes resulting from the use of this material. While every attempt has been made to provide information that is both accurate and effective, the author does not assume any responsibility for the accuracy or use/misuse of this information.

SUMMARY

Special thanks to www.anykindapills.com team for their endless support, my partner AJG in London for editing this E-book, to Sereine and Lucie Bale for believing in me, to my parents and family members for their love.

CHAPTER1

IS EXERCISE THE BEST FAT BURNER?

I will start this book with direct strong words, exercising doesn't always make you lose weight subscribing to a gym club, pushing hard to lose extra weight, various studies demonstrates the small impact of weight lost by exercising.

Almost daily you hear women talking or complaining about their weight, they need to get off the extra pounds. Over time without the knowledge knowing the metabolism of their body, people in vain try dieting and eating the wrong food. Every day men and woman subscribe for gym clubs. The wealthiest have personal coaches, it becomes like surviving a navy seal cut, running, weight lifting, military exercises. All this without counting long walks, swimming like dolphins and running like Forest Gump. After all this gym lovers should have muscles of Hercules with the strength of superman and their eating healthy like an athlete but unexpectedly are keeping the extra weight. By frustration women tend to fraction their meals consequently lose a lot of muscles, energy, and then the metabolism system suffers. The fat remains, why? This is unfair? They are doing everything in the book but the extra is there, not leaving at all. Curious, mystery, frustration, how to lose the overweight?

Losing weight is a commitment with a huge focus. Reaching your ideal shape will need you to input a lot of physical and mental effort. Consider all the hours spent on your bed, sofa and eating what you should never have as pay back for your body. Re member all the adverts seen on TV, heard on the radio or claimed by notorious doctors preaching the only effective way of losing the extra pounds and have an Olympic body is only through exercising. Is this the truth?

Understanding the basics on how a person can gain or lose weight is very important. You eat and gain calories or energy for your body that is what help us move around, go shopping, drive a car, travelling. The more calories you store the more movement you will need to do. By consuming more calories or energy then needed it will turn into fat. In conclusion the energy you don't burn off stocks as fat by your body. According to nutritionist DR Susan Jebb, head of nutrition and Health research at Medical Research Council and one of US government's consultants in various dietary programme thinks you have to go beyond exercising. For instant 4 hours of cycling will help you burn off 1000 calories and this represents 4 burgers only.   I think the situation seems more realistic, easier to get the body shape and to maintain it when you are in your 20's but in your 40's it takes a lot of commitment and a lot more of exercise.

The best way to look slimmer isn't by exercising, unless you are willing to spend money. Take in consideration the numerous gym hours and long exhausting programmes that are available. Professor Paul Gately of the Carnegie Weight Management Institution in Leeds based in the UK. He estimated to be able to lose a pound of body fat you must run a marathon about 73 Miles and by skipping a meal a day for a week will give the same results. Now you realise with less effort and mental focus you can achieve the same results. Another convincing study comes from Dr Timothy Church from University of Louisiana; he compared for six months four groups of overweight woman. 3 groups respectively exercise 72,136 and 194 minutes for a week. The fourth and last group followed a diet programme without exercising.

In this study, Church wanted to demonstrate the theory of compensation, the woman who exercised dearly in the first three groups didn't lose that much weight and some of them even gain more than before. They never changed their eating habits and we all know after a good workout your body naturally will want to replace the energy burn off by eating.

Steven Gortmaker and Kendrin Sonneville backed up Church conclusions. Gortmaker and Kendrin studied for 18 months the concept of energy gap. Energy gap is the imbalance of energy taken and spent by human body. These great scientists were able to demonstrate the energy spent is replaced by a greater amount through eating.

Where does this idea of exercise come from to make you believe you can easily lose weight? Jean Mayer a French-American was able to make apparent the link between exercise and weight loss. Scientists adopted the idea without providing proof to back it up. Mayer's study was based on rats, babies and school girls. The theory was less energy you burned the more likely it will turn into fat. Mayer was a son of two well-known physiologists and a World War II hero, as a nutritionist he became a major voice in public health issues. He was an advisor to the white house and World Health Organisation, he changed people's thinking by promoting his study and vision, exercise and fitness are the only way to lose fat. Working out, being Slimmer, back then in the 60's and 70's he became a symbol of healthy living. He needed to convince various entrepreneurs on the potential of this huge market and governments saw new tax incomes for the treasury.

Mayer's studies on rats, babies and young school girls demonstrated that less active subjects were the more likely to gain weight. In other terms the less active you are the most likely to get fat. Son of world hero, Mayer easily became a leading nutritionist and an important voice in a scientific community in public heath matter. Also, He built a bridge between fitness and exercise by using his role as an advisor to the white house and World Health Organisation. During the 60s and 70s his ideas spread all over western civilization and became pandemic. Populations wanted to be fit, have muscular bodies and this became referential for healthy living. The entrepreneur eagle eyes saw opportunity to make money.

The Generation who came after World War II were mostly peaceful, conservative and living close to industries. People were sedentary, people ate distortedly and obesity stroked in the population. Now Paediatrics clinics are recording a great number of type II diabetes, these kind of alarming statics were found in geriatrics wards, three in five need to lose their pork fat. Why nobody is stopping it? We are more focus on eliminating the symptoms instead of going to the root of the problem.

Since when have we stopped applying basic logic? Remember in science or philosophy class we solve problems by observing, finding the cause and the effects. A well-known professor of endocrinology and metabolism at a Medical School in Plymouth, Terry Wilkin believes we get confused between cause and effects. One of his famous researches was on obesity "Fatness leads to inactivity, but inactivity do not lead to fatness". This study was based on children and Wilkin studied their health for 11 years by observing the weight and activity from the age of 5 to 16. At the end of the study, when comparing the body mass of active children with less active ones, guess what? There was no significant difference on body fat. In other words the 300 subject proved that exercise is not making the children lose weight. That's why the heavy calorific food industry doesn't worry about government sponsored programmes that primarily focus on exercises instead of foods.

Wilkin and Church studies demonstrated human beings tend to reward themselves with food. Wilkin study was based on school girls with accelerometers on them. He separated the girls into two groups. The first group had 1.7 hours a week of physical activity. When the girls went home they did the reverse. At the end Wilkins came to the conclusion that the physical activity was controlled by the brain and not by the environment

In conclusion, your environment will do little in your fight against obesity, physical education; extra professional activity, friends and family encouragement are less influential on what exercise we will do. Physical activity helps regulate your energy expenditure.

Obesity expert's world was shocked by Wilkins findings and rebuked it without any proof. Dr Ken Fox, professor of exercise and health science at Bristol University and advisor to government on obesity strategy, thinks this study has created controversy because it was the first of kind on children. He adds it's too early to start discarding physical activity and all paper works done on the importance of it. "Terry's point is right," says Paul Gately, "but it's not right in the context of public health promotion. In people who have lost weight and kept weight off, physical activity is almost always involved. And those people who just do diet are more likely to fail, as are those who just do exercise. You need a combination of the two, because we're talking about human beings, not machines. We know that dietary behaviour is quite a negative behaviour – we have to deny ourselves something. There aren't any diets out there that people enjoy. But people do enjoy being physically active.

Jebb backs DR ken Fox way of thinking by saying "What we want to avoid is people thinking they can control their weight simply by dieting," adds Jebb, this will encourage anorexia in teenage girls and just controlling your food won't be the healthiest way to live, Weightwatchers and Slimming world integrates exercises in their diet programmes. Scientific study demonstrated exercise is an important element in preventing weight gain.

Overweight people find it very hard to exercise; eating just over 100 calories a day can increase your weight by 10 pound a year. I totally agree with Wilkin when he thinks education is must come first and eating habits must change to lower energy calorie intake, lower body weight will help us spend more energy or do more activity. I would love to see higher tax on junk food, on tobacco and lower prices on healthy low sugar food.

Governments in various countries refuse to take bold action to change people habits because of the economic consequences. Anne Milton minister for public health thinks "There's not a magic bullet here," she says. "Despite the best efforts of government actually the public's health hasn't improved hugely.Change4Life government's programme for healthy living is doing well but not enough.

Junk food still has a comfortable life in our economy, Secretary of state for Health Andrew Lansley and Milton wants to work with the industry. When it comes to food the best strategy is to change habits and the amount of food types we consume.

RUNNING ON EMPTY: IS FAT A FEMINE ISSUE?

I couldn't start talking about diet without clarifying this issue new scientific research from US tends to show the low influence of intense workout in weight loss compared to normal workout practice in many Gyms. Barry Braun, an associate professor of kinesiology at University of Massachusetts, thinks exercise in low intensity such as walking will help in burning calories. His studies in this will not trigger the calorie compensation proven by Church and Wilkin. Braun showed by standing you burn more energy than by sitting without increasing the appetite hormones in your blood.

Scientific studies prove that women bodies can easily store fat better than men. Now we can understand why a multi-billion weight-loss industry is strictly mainly targeting woman. To prove this Braun simply put overweight women and man on treadmills for certain periods of time. Women's blood levels of insulin decreased while appetite hormones increased, while nothing happened to the men. Professor Ken Fox specialist of exercise and health science agrees that it is tougher for women to lose weight than for men.

CHAPTER 2

DIFFERENT TYPE OF DIETS

DO YOU KNOW DETOX DIET?

Do you believe in them? The aim of detox diet is to clean your body from toxins. Some Doctors are suspecting detox diet might be too risky with great consequences on your health. Detox diet is quiet popular and before you do decide you should read this first.

How good does detox diet works? You can lose weight on detox diet because of they are very low on calories. Unless you are sick, biologists never agreed with the idea that your body needs help to get rid of toxins. Doctor Frank Sacks of Harvard School of Public Health declares that our organs and immune system function properly when it comes to eliminating toxins.

People follow different detox diet, they are a huge range of them, some of them implicates fasting, or consuming liquids with some food or not, with fruits and vegetables. Detox diets are not sustainable in a long term.

Detox diets will make you feel weak and hungry and no assurance to feel healthy. Low calories and poor nutrients can weaken people with a possible chance of side effects such as low energy, low blood sugar, muscle aches, fatigue, feeling dizzy or lightheaded and nausea.

These are recommended foods vegetables, fruits, whole grains, lean protein and whole foods. If you are planning to lose weight avoid processed food. Detox diet works better with a specific exercise habit. By combining a detox diet with exercise you will most likely increase the effect.

You must remember detox diets have great limitations, a cycle of eating certain food types, constantly checking your calories and maintaining shopping lists. For example detox diet can be herbal, pills, powders, enemas, dry fruits, seeds and nuts.

Detox is a low energy consumption diet, you might not have enough strength to maintain your exercise habits and you might need to reconsider your budget, supplements are quiet costly and you can easily purchase most of the items online. Alternative solution try a blender, easy receipts makes nutritional drinks.

CHAPTER 3

LOW FAT DIET, DOES IT WORK?

For decades low fat diet has been promoted as a solution for losing weight, as a way to prevent and control heart diseases and other diseases related to weight problem like blood pressure. Even the food industry went through a huge change by creating low fat products. Lowering the fat in goods changed the taste which affected sales. Like a bad Chef the food industry resolved this huge problem by increasing the amount of sugar or and salt. By Refining the grains sometimes by adding preservatives with other chemicals helped to regenerate new products. Guess what? With nice marketing receipts all sales went back up it worked.

Why is the number of obesity still increasing? Why weight control is becoming an obsession for both men and women?

Statistics shows that 45% of Americans calories come from fat and oils, 13% of adults were obese with a critical weight control problem and 1% had type II diabetes. With 33% of Americans intake their calories from oils and fat. Hence, the number of adult's obesity dangerously moves up to 34% and sadly the number of adults with diabetes rose up to 11%.

I can imagine the next question, why lowering fat by the food industry didn't create the effect expected? Various nutritional studies demonstrate that the total amount of fat in a diet isn't really related to the weight or diseases. Today you are going to discover one of the hidden secrets from the general population from the gym and food industries, what is important is the type of fat and the amount of calories in a diet.

Which fat is good for your body? It's simple, bad fats, hydrogenation or artificial trans-fat are called saturated fats. They are risky and deadly, they can increase the risk of huge list of diseases. You will find them in cakes, biscuits or in processed foods. They are also naturally found in low levels in meat and dairy food.

Dr Charles Livingston in DC, is an expert of liver performance, has highlighted food reputed healthy like chicken noodles and others contains monosodium glutamate or concentrated salt, this can lead to weight gain and cause headaches, asthma attacks and other illness. Additionally, low calories breakfast meals such as Kellogs special K, salad dressing like Ranch, breakfast bars such as Balance or Power bar have HFCS. High Fructose Corn Syrup also used in soft drinks, it brings sweetness to our aliment. This sugary liquid goes straight into your liver and prevents your pancreas from producing insulin. Also, tricks your brain to never feeling full. Today you can easily understand the most likely origin of belly fat on man or menopause belly in woman called estrogen fat affecting various diet programmes. You lose weight and after a while gain back the belly or hips fat. A nice diet should be able to increase your liver performance, this organ breakdown fats, sugar and filter toxins.

Good fats also called monounsaturated and polyunsaturated fats, they are good for the heart and body. Most of the fat you eat should come from unsaturated source or monounsaturated and polyunsaturated fats. You will find good fats in nuts, vegetables oil and fish

Monounsaturated Fat Sources	Omega-6 Polyunsaturated Fat Sources	Omega-3 Polyunsaturated Fat Sources
Nuts Vegetable oils Canola oil Olive oil High oleic safflower oil Sunflower oil Avocado	Soybean oil Corn oil Safflower oil	Soybean oil Canola oil Walnuts Flaxseed Fish: trout, herring, and salmon

Low fat diets generically stops people eating good fats for your body. Generally a carbohydrate replaces fat suppression in people diets programmes. Most people replace it on aliments like white bread, white rice, potatoes and sugary drinks. Sometimes people replace it by low fat or fat free products which use a great amount of sugar, salt or refined carbohydrates. High blood sugar and great level of insulin are caused by huge levels of carbohydrates entering your liver and blocking your pancreas normal activities. Increasing the intake of carbohydrates on a long period of time can increase the risk of heart disease and diabetes like you were eating saturated fat.

A good diet doesn't replace bad fat by carbohydrates but by good fat.

CHAPTER 4

HOW YOUR BODY PROCESSES FAT IN YOUR BLOODSTREAM?

Fat mixed in a diet can increase cholesterol in the bloodstream far more than cholesterol in food does. We are not going to argue that all foods contain a certain quantity of fat. A vegetable like carrots and lettuce are quintessential reputed fat free still contains a small amount of this element. That is the way nature demonstrates the important of this nutriment. Without fat we have no energy to burn and our body cannot store energy. Fat is an important part for cell membranes helping to manage what comes in and out.

Cholesterol is a key element in the making of estrogen, testosterone and vitamin D and in other vital compositions. Fats are highly influential in molecules that can direct the way muscles respond to insulin. You might not know but fat can increase or decrease an inflammation.

Lipoproteins, high- Lipoproteins are the fruit of the inability of blood and water to eliminate fat. Storing fat in the blood is the way that your body is programmed, lipoproteins can carry little fat, mix with blood and as a protein it flows. Sometimes they are big and stuffy, other small and dense, triglycerides, density lipoproteins.

Low density lipoproteins (LDL) is a transporter, it takes your cholesterol from the liver to the rest of the body. LDL delivers fat to all your cells and when it has too many the particles are simply deposited in your coronary arteries and other arteries. It's like your sink pipe the more rubbish or food left in your plates during the washing the more likely it will obstruct the water passage. The more fat deposited by the LDL in your arteries the more difficulty your blood will flow through your heart. The deposit can form plaque that can break and obstruct your arteries then cause a heart attack or stroke. Bad cholesterol or plaques are very harmful or deadly.

Where does go the good fat? HDL, high density lipoproteins farms cholesterol from LDL, bloodstream and from arteries then deposit all into the Liver. The liver breaks down all collections for disposal. HDL cleans your bloodstream and it's considered as good cholesterol. Various diets are available for LDL reductions and increase your HDL.

CHAPTER 5

CHOLESTEROL LEVELS ARE AFFECTED BY FOOD

The food intake determines the type of fat you will find in a bloodstream. In other words, HDL and LDL cholesterol levels in your bloodstream are greatly influence by your diet. Levels and type of carbohydrate play it's a lot HDL and LDL levels hence let us not forget cholesterol level s in a food still plays a small role.

Unsaturated fats, good fat have a great effect on improving cholesterol levels, heart performance and many other roles that we cannot listed and we leave that to cardiologist. Nuts, vegetable oils, plants and seeds are containing great amount of unsaturated fats.

Let us dig a little bit more on good fats; they are two types of unsaturated fats, monounsaturated and polyunsaturated fats.

Monounsaturated fats are found in high levels in olives, peanut, canola, avocados, hazelnuts, pecans, almonds, nuts, pumpkin, sesame and seeds. Polyunsaturated fats are in great levels in sunflower, corn, soybean, flaxseed oils, walnuts, flax seeds, fish and canola oil. These aliments have a great amount of both fats.

Omega-3 fats belongs to polyunsaturated fats group and it's one of the dearest fat of the supplement industry, naturally not produce by your body but found in foods like fish to be eaten 3 times a week, plants, chia seeds, flax seeds, walnuts, oil like flaxseed, canola and soybean.

CHAPTER 6

HOW CARBOHYDRATES DOES EFFECTS CHOLESTEROL LEVELS?

A great Dutch research team ran 60 analysis trials that examined the effects of carbohydrates and other fats on blood levels. A group consumed good fats instead of carbohydrates and LDL were deceased in the bloodstream. Naturally the HDL increased and protected the heart. Optimal Macronutrient is a random intake trial ran by Heart Health (Omni heart), by replacing a rich carbohydrate diet by a rich unsaturated fat diet decreased blood pressure, improved lipid levels and reduces LDL levels.

Governments and health officials do not have a strict guide line to protect the populations, to make sure unsaturated fats are greatly consume. The American heart association carefully estimated 8 to 10 percent of calories are from unsaturated fats. Hence, 30% of Greeks following traditional diets mostly consumed polyunsaturated and monounsaturated fats from olive oil.

It's hard to eat and to count how many bad and good fat you are taking. One rule prevails; learn to choose food rich in unsaturated fats.

More than 50 years ago research showed a relation between high blood cholesterol levels with increased risk for heart disease. The aim was to warn about food that contains cholesterol like eggs and liver. Most people produce more cholesterol than they consume from their food. Numerous studies demonstrated a light relation between the amounts of cholesterol a person eat from food and his or her blood cholesterol levels but important for heart disease.

Another was on 80,000 female nurses by Harvard researchers found that eating an egg a day wasn't associated with heart disease. Scientist thought that the great amount of nutrient in eggs counter balance the increase in risk of heart disease. In the same study, on diabetes patient had a reverse effect by eating eggs daily increased risks of heart disease.

Moderate consumption of eggs on none diabetes man and woman can be part of a healthy diet, this research doesn't recommend a daily omelette especially for diabetes and heart diseases patient.

The majority of the population have a higher level of cholesterol than the one eaten through food. Avoiding cholesterol rich foods can reduce LDL levels.

CHAPTER 7

ARE SATURATED FATS REALLY ONLY BAD FOR YOU?

Atkins diet deliberating avoiding carbohydrates but includes high saturated fats like bacon, butter, steak, cheese and other similar foods. Over the decades controversial debates are heating the nutritionist science community about how bad are saturated fat is for the body. That is why Atkins diet has been an atomic bomb; recent studies are backing up Atkins theory suggesting eating saturated does not automatically drives up the risk of heart disease. Another stunning 21 studies of 350000 people analysing tem for 23 years, the scientist tried to find a correlation between saturated fat consumed and coronary heart disease (CHD), stroke and Cardiovascular disease (CVD). The epidemiologist report was incredible, from an epidemiologic view the evidence are not inconclusive or insufficient on the correlation between saturated fat and CVD, stroke and CHD.

Journalist founded the scoop of the year, as usual they quickly jumped into to conclusions, scientists just declared saturated fat is not responsible for heart diseases, some blogs validating saturated fats has healthy and scientist have declared bacon, butter and cheese as healthy. Journalist naturally made it look simple. No insufficient evidence does mean you are not guilty; wrongly interpreting conclusions can cause deadly habits. By reading the full study report, the general conclusion seems to be clear, replacing saturated fats by polyunsaturated and monounsaturated fats lowers LDL levels and increases HDL cholesterols levels, can help to prevent insulin resistance, prevention against diabetes.

Maybe by now you have understood the key message of this chapter, learning and understanding this key message will help you break a myth shared by a great portion of the world population, cutting down on saturated fat isn't beneficiary unless you replace it with saturated fat with refined carbohydrates like white bread, white rice, nice English mashed potatoes, sugary drinks and similar aliment. Minimizing saturated fat consummation and choosing to eat refined carbohydrates in place lowers LDL cholesterol and HDL levels and increases triglycerides. This is like eating saturated fat only and this is not recommendable to insulin resistance patient because they are overweight or inactive.

The latest American dietary guidelines report recommends getting less than 10% of calories each day from saturated fat, the American Heart Association was more hard dropping the percentage of saturated fat to 7%. I think the majority of our population will agree that reducing your diet into percentage is not practical at all. When a common man or woman eats, they do not thing in term of percentage of fat intake in a day. Once a humane being feels hungry they think on terms of eating food and not nutrient.

The average American has various saturated fat sources and the most used is pizza with cheese, other dairy products like whole or reduced fat milk, butter, dairy desserts and meat like sausage, bacon, beef and hamburgers. Cookies, grains based desserts and Mexican dishes are also a great source of fat. Keep in mind all foods contains fats, good or bad, this might surprise some people but chicken and nuts have saturated fat even though they are at lower levels compared to beef, cheese and ice cream. Some oil or fruits have high levels of saturated fats for instance coconut, coconut oil, palm oil highly used by the food industry and palm kernel oil.

The main rule to a healthy diet is to always keep your saturated fat as low as possible, it's almost impossible to completely eliminate saturated fats from a healthy diet because healthy food like olive oil, walnuts, salmon and other fishes also have saturated fat but at a low levels. It will be not recommendable to cut down on nuts, oils, and fish to eliminate saturated fat. As you read previously red meat and fat dairy products for example cheese, milk, ice cream, butter have high levels of fat that you must reduce and replace it by healthy fats like fish, nuts, seeds, plant oils, avocadoes and avoid food that are high in refined carbohydrates.

CHAPTER 8

TRANS-FATS

Trans fatty acids is obtained by a process called hydrogenation, this consist of heating vegetable oils in the presence of hydrogen gas and a catalyst. Trans fatty are well known under the name trans-fats. Hydrogenating vegetable oils stables the oil; makes it solid and easy for transportation. Also, hydrogenating oil is an economic and easy to utilise. Hydrogenating vegetable oil can allow repeated heating without breaking down like oils you found in fast foods, Kebabs, burgers or other frying fast foods. Hydrogenated oils are like a saturated fat you will find it in baked foods, margarines and food industry. Another great study was conducted by the Nurses Health on the effect of margarine on women. 50% greater risk of heart disease of the participant who ate 4 teaspoons of margarine compare to women who ate rarely margarine.

Also hydrogenating oil is an economic and easy to utilise. Hydrogenating vegetable oil can allow repeated heating without breaking down like oils you found in fast foods, Kebabs, burgers or other frying fast foods. Hydrogenated oils are like a saturated fat you will find it in baked foods, margarines and used within the food industry. Another great study was conducted by the Nurses Health on the effect of margarine on women. 50% greater risk of heart disease of the participant who ate 4 teaspoons of margarine compare to women who ate rarely margarine.

So should we try preferring butter over margarine? No, there are other alternatives butter and margarine both use vegetable oil and a best alternative can be olive oil, canola or other less harmful vegetable oil with a buttery flavour. You still not convinced? You could choose soft margarine with trans-fat free and low on saturated fat. Now days we can easily find none expensive from healthy oils, trans-fat free with cholesterol lowering benefits. You will need to eat two servings a day to lower your bad Cholesterol. Trans-Fat can also be naturally found in beef fat and dairy fat in low levels

Trans-fats have a much devastating effect on cholesterol level compared to saturated fats. They always raise LDL level and decrease HDL levels. They fire up through inflammations various diseases like stroke, heart disease, diabetes and other life threatening chronic conditions, affecting the immune system activity, contributing to insulin resistance. By removing trans- fat produce by the food industry in U.S. will prevent 6 to 19 percent of heart attacks and related deaths, this means 200,000 more people living longer and savings for the health care system. Trans-fat is so bad eve n a tiny quantity in the diet can be deadly; by consuming 2 percent of calories from trans- fat daily increases the risk of coronary heart disease by 23 percent.

Research ran in 1990's demonstrated commercially baked goods, margarines, snack foods, processed foods, French fries, other fried foods prepared in restaurants, fast food franchises were the daily source of six grams of trans-fat for Americans. Knowing the effects of trans-fat on the body I would prefer it was zero percent.

U.S. government timidly reacted by publishing a law' forcing the food industry to label trans-fats and trans-reduce fats. This pushed big brands to use trans-free oils and fats in their products. The affect was beneficial, for disease control and prevention finds published a report stating that the level of trans-fat in the blood of Americans dropped from 58 percent in 2000 to 2009 proof of the effect of the law. Ideally by eliminating trans-fat in all commercialise foods and snacks would had a greater impact on the population and on the health care bill.

Some experts feared the industry would replace trans-fats by saturated fats but a 2010 survey showed 83% of major grocery store Brand in the food industry and restaurant dishes reduced trans-fat without increasing saturated fats.

While Trans-fat is losing grounds in developed countries but it rising at phenomena speed in developing countries. Cheap hydrogenated soybean oil is not only used in the industries but for home cooking also. Changing local traditional oils towards trans-rich partially hydrogenated oils has raised cardiovascular disease at epidemic levels never seen on developing countries.

CHAPTER 9

FATS AND CANCERS

I needed to break another myth in this book. So far, no association between dietary and certain cancers, any link or evidence were found between fat and cancer cell or cancer risk.

Where this myth does came from? Back in 1980's, dietary experts believed fat was one of the major cause of breast Cancer. This research was based on simple international statistics comparisons showing higher breast cancer rate in countries with higher fat intake. Further study were done throughout the decades and concluded they were no links between fats and certain cancer risk or diseases. The Women's Health Initiative dietary Modification Trial was responsible for the study of low fat diet on developing cancer breasts compared to regular diet end up with the same results. The National Institutes of Health ran a study found a light link between fat and postmenopausal breast cancer and fat, after various studies all suspicions fall. Harvard researchers failed to find a link between breast cancer and different types of fats. Some evidences are driving studies towards animal fat consume at a younger age.

Women who ate diets in high animal fats had 40 to 50 percent higher risk of breast cancer, this study from Nurses' Health Study II, suggested the meat may contain other elements such as hormones. Another study done in Europe Union suggested a lower risk of breast cancer among women consuming monounsaturated fats in form of olive oil.

Same processes were run with studies regarding colon cancer. International comparisons like in breast cancer between dietary fat intake colon cancer risk. These early finding were found to be false and revealed instead a weak correlation. Women's Health Initiative Dietary Modification Trial who ate low fat diet developed colon cancer at the same level as women who did not. Some research highlighted a great number of evidence that high intake of red meat like beef, pork , lamb, and processed meat like hot dogs, bacon, sausage and deli meats does increase colon cancer risk. It's recommended to avoid processed meat at all cost and to limit red meat intake at 2 twice a week.

Prostate cancer was studied too; no evidence supported any links between fats and the risk of prostate cancer. Hence evidence supported diets high in animal fat and saturated fat increase prostate cancer risk. Some studies are contradicting these findings, others are accusing unsaturated fats and we all can agreed on the need of further research on this deadly disease.

Much more research needs to be done on the type of all cancers, Harvard researchers in the Nurses' Health Study found a link between trans-fats with the risk for non-Hodgkin's lymphoma.

CHAPTER 10

RELATION BETWEEN CHRONIC CONDITIONS AND DIETARY FATS

A great amount of researches were conducted on the effects of fats heart disease and more are needed. More and more studies are being published on the influence of dietary fats on depression, osteoporosis, age memory loss, cognitive decline, muscular degeneration, multiple sclerosis, infertility and endometriosis and many other chronic diseases. These early findings remains insufficient to provide significant evident or guidelines. At the moment we can only theorize and suggest or recommend.

Dietary fats and Obesity

For decades, the nutritionist believed the more fat you eat the more weight you gain. Countless studies have countered and eliminated this myth or theory, which replaced fat by carbohydrate intake. The idea that food intake equals body fat is not exactly true;

this was misleading the general population. Over the years the Americans have reduced calories portion intake but the portion of obesity keeps on growing at an alarming rate.

Any diet that helps you take lower calories works only over a short period, a low fat diet can lead to weight loss over a short period same when following high-fat, low carbohydrate diet or a high-protein, low-carbohydrate diet. This was demonstrated in the Women's Health Initiative Dietary Modification Trial. The Participants were following a low fat diet and for a long period of time. At end, they did not lose or gain weight, they were more like a person following usual diet. Another great research comparing numerous weight loss strategies concluded that Mediterranean, low-fat and low-carbohydrate diets performed at same results and at the same speed. In a different study Mediterranean diet was performing better than low-fat diet.

Your diet quality is very important on preventing various diseases like heart disease, they ability to keep the weight off is important. A 120000 study for 20 years of men and women by Harvard School of Public Health evaluated the influence of small changes on weight gain. The participants were separated onto 3 groups, the first group ate more nuts, high-fat food that was forbidden for dieters, gained less weight during the study and they gain about a half of pound every four years. The second group ate more vegetables, whole grains, fruits and gained less. Hence, the third group ate more red meat and processed meat, during the study they gained more weight than any participants in other groups, almost more than a pound every four years.3.4,1.3,1.0 and 0.6 pounds every four years were respectively the pounds gained by the third group eating fries, potatoes and potato chips, sugary drinks and refined grains. Vegetables, nuts, fruits, whole grain calories increase in the body and eliminate other foods calories.

Before we conclude, I just wanted to say I'm really sorry you were a victim of lobbies. Yes, exercise has an impact on your body but just a little. Increasing number of new research in the U.S and UK demonstrates the tiny influence of exercise on your weight lost problems. Remember back in the 80's and 90's people used to receive as a gift a gym club membership card and wear colourful nylon sportswear then massively go to different aerobics class? Where are all these aerobics TV shows that all big channels used to broadcast? Why it's disappearing?

United Kingdom and United state studies both demonstrate you have a long way to that nice looking great body. Is it worthless to spend so much money on gym membership? In US a not-profit clinical research has been conducted by the Mayo Clinic. The conclusion of this study was shocking, exercise alone had a very modest impact on short term goals when it comes to weight loss compare to scientific dietary program. This is a scientific discovery, scary for the sports industry. It sounds unbelievable but we are talking about the sporting goods market, in the United States experts projected 63 million US dollars in 2014. This figure doesn't corporate 25 to 30 billion U.S dollars consumer purchases on recreational transportation items such as bicycles, pleasures boats, RVs and snowmobiles. Now we can easily understand why medical professionals are suffering pressures for all kinds of lobbies and governments don't want to lose their taxes income or don't want to see more people losing jobs. Sporting goods market has multiple aspects to it such as export, job statics and a lot more. Let's come back to our subject. Exercise is good for us but it won't help a lot when it comes to losing weight

Many more studies need to be conducted before any official recommendation from nutritionist experts are published but we can agree on a choice of a healthy diet such as described by www.anykindapills.com . Registering and following free advices of www.anykindapills.com will help you stay healthy. Remember the amount of food you eat will help you burn calories, eat more unsaturated fats, will help you more to maintain or lose weight.

REFERENCES

1. USDA Center for Nutrition Policy and Promotion. Nutrition Insights: Insight 5: Is Total Fat Consumption Really Decreasing? In; 1998.

2. Flegal K, Carroll M, Kuczmarski R, Johnson C. Overweight and obesity in the United States: prevalence and trends, 1960-1994. *Int J ObesRelatMetabDisord*. 1998;22:39-47.

3. Diabetes in America, 2nd Edition. Bethesda, MD: National Institute of Health Publication; 1995.

4. Wright JD, Wang, C-Y. *Trends in intake of energy and macronutrients in adults from 1999-2000 through 2007-2008*. Hyattsville, MD: National Center for Health Statistics; 2010.

5. Flegal KM, Carroll MD, Ogden CL, Curtin LR. Prevalence and trends in obesity among US adults, 1999-2008. *JAMA*. 2010;303:235-41.

6. Centers for Disease Control and Prevention. National diabetes fact sheet: national estimates and general information on diabetes and prediabetes in the United States, 2011. U.S. Dept. of Health and Human Services, 2011. Accessed January 11, 2012.

7. Appel L, Sacks F, Carey V, et al. Effects of protein, monounsaturated fat, and carbohydrate intake on blood pressure and serum lipids: results of the OmniHeart randomized trial. *JAMA*. 2005;294:2455-64

8. Beresford S, Johnson K, Ritenbaugh C, et al. Low-fat dietary pattern and risk of colorectal cancer: the Women's Health

Initiative Randomized Controlled Dietary Modification Trial. *JAMA*. 2006;295:643-54.

9. Howard B, Manson J, Stefanick M, et al. Low-fat dietary pattern and weight change over 7 years: the Women's Health Initiative Dietary Modification Trial. *JAMA*. 2006;295:39-49.

10. Howard B, Van Horn L, Hsia J, et al. Low-fat dietary pattern and risk of cardiovascular disease: the Women's Health Initiative Randomized Controlled Dietary Modification Trial. *JAMA*. 2006;295:655-66.

11. Mente A, de Koning L, Shannon HS, Anand SS. A systematic review of the evidence supporting a causal link between dietary factors and coronary heart disease. *Arch Intern Med*. 2009;169:659-69.

12. Sacks FM, Bray GA, Carey VJ, et al. Comparison of weight-loss diets with different compositions of fat, protein, and carbohydrates. *N Engl J Med*. 2009;360:859-73.

13. Mozaffarian D, Micha R, Wallace S. Effects on coronary heart disease of increasing polyunsaturated fat in place of saturated fat: a systematic review and meta-analysis of randomized controlled trials. *PLoS Med*. 2010;7:e1000252.

14. Mozaffarian D, Hao T, Rimm EB, Willett WC, Hu FB. Changes in diet and lifestyle and long-term weight gain in women and men. *N Engl J Med*. 2011;364:2392-404.

15. Hooper L, Summerbell CD, Thompson R, et al. Reduced or modified dietary fat for preventing cardiovascular disease. *Cochrane Database Syst Rev*. 2011:CD002137.

16. Siri-Tarino PW, Sun Q, Hu FB, Krauss RM. Saturated fatty acids and risk of coronary heart disease: modulation by replacement nutrients. *CurrAtheroscler Rep*. 2010;12:384-90.

17. Hu FB. Are refined carbohydrates worse than saturated fat? *Am J ClinNutr*. 2010;91:1541-2.

18. Jakobsen MU, Dethlefsen C, Joensen AM, et al. Intake of carbohydrates compared with intake of saturated fatty acids and risk of myocardial infarction: importance of the glycemic index. *Am J ClinNutr*. 2010;91:1764-8.

19. Mensink R, Zock P, Kester A, Katan M. Effects of dietary fatty acids and carbohydrates on the ratio of serum total to HDL cholesterol and on serum lipids and apolipoproteins: a meta-analysis of 60 controlled trials. *Am J ClinNutr*. 2003;77:1146-55.

20. Taubes G. What if It's All Been a Big Fat Lie? *The New York Times*, July 7, 2002.

21. Siri-Tarino PW, Sun Q, Hu FB, Krauss RM. Meta-analysis of prospective cohort studies evaluating the association of saturated fat with cardiovascular disease. *Am J ClinNutr*. 2010;91:535-46.

22. Micha R, Mozaffarian D. Saturated fat and cardiometabolic risk factors, coronary heart disease, stroke, and diabetes: a fresh look at the evidence. *Lipids*. 2010;45:893-905.

23. Beck L. Saturated Fat Is Not Your Heart's Enemy. The Globe and Mail 2010.

24. Moore J. NOT GUILTY: The Long-Standing Vilification of Saturated Fat Finally Turning to Vindication. 2010. Accessed January 11, 2012.

25. Astrup A, Dyerberg J, Elwood P, et al. The role of reducing intakes of saturated fat in the prevention of cardiovascular disease: where does the evidence stand in 2010? *Am J ClinNutr*. 2011;93:684-8.

26. Riserus U, Willett WC, Hu FB. Dietary fats and prevention of type 2 diabetes. *Prog Lipid Res*. 2009;48:44-51.

27. U.S. Department of Agriculture, U.S. Department of Health and Human Services. *Dietary Guidelines for Americans, 2010*. Washington, D.C.: U.S. Government Printing Office; 2010.

28. Lichtenstein AH, Appel LJ, Brands M, et al. Diet and lifestyle recommendations revision 2006: a scientific statement from the American Heart Association Nutrition Committee. *Circulation*. 2006;114:82-96.

29. National Cancer Institute. Risk Factor Monitoring and Methods: Table 1. Top Food Sources of Saturated Fat among U.S. Population, 2005–2006. *NHANES*.Accessed January 11, 2012.

30. Mozaffarian D, Pischon T, Hankinson S, et al. Dietary intake of trans fatty acids and systemic inflammation in women. *Am J ClinNutr*. 2004;79:606-12.

31. Mozaffarian D, Katan M, Ascherio A, Stampfer M, Willett W. Trans fatty acids and cardiovascular disease. *N Engl J Med*. 2006;354:1601-13.

32. Allison DB, Egan SK, Barraj LM, Caughman C, Infante M, Heimbach JT. Estimated intakes of trans fatty and other fatty acids in the U.S. population. *J Am Diet Assoc*. 1999;99:166-74.

33. Mozaffarian D, Jacobson MF, Greenstein JS. Food reformulations to reduce trans fatty acids. *N Engl J Med*. 2010;362:2037-9.

34. Kratz M. Dietary cholesterol, atherosclerosis and coronary heart disease. *HandbExpPharmacol*. 2005:195-213.

35. Hu F, Stampfer M, Rimm E, et al. A prospective study of egg consumption and risk of cardiovascular disease in men and women. *JAMA*. 1999;281:1387-94.

36. Hu F, Stampfer M, Manson J, et al. Dietary fat intake and the risk of coronary heart disease in women.*NEngl J Med*. 1997;337:1491-9.

37. Fernandez M. Dietary cholesterol provided by eggs and plasma lipoproteins in healthy populations.*CurrOpinClinNutrMetab Care*. 2006;9:8-12.

38. Willett WC. *Nutritional Epidemiology*. New York: Oxford University Press; 1998.

39. Ascherio A, Rimm E, Giovannucci E, Spiegelman D, Stampfer M, Willett W. Dietary fat and risk of coronary heart disease in men: cohort follow up study in the United States. *BMJ*. 1996;313:84-90.

40. Hu F, Manson J, Willett W. Types of dietary fat and risk of coronary heart disease: a critical review. *J Am CollNutr*. 2001;20:5-19.

41. Fung TT, Rexrode KM, Mantzoros CS, Manson JE, Willett WC, Hu FB. Mediterranean diet and incidence of and mortality from coronary heart disease and stroke in women. *Circulation*. 2009;119:1093-100.

42. Kastorini CM, Milionis HJ, Esposito K, Giugliano D, Goudevenos JA, Panagiotakos DB. The effect of Mediterranean diet on metabolic syndrome and its components: a meta-analysis of 50 studies and 534,906 individuals. *J Am CollCardiol*. 2011;57:1299-313.

43. Kaushik M, Mozaffarian D, Spiegelman D, Manson JE, Willett WC, Hu FB. Long-chain omega-3 fatty acids, fish intake, and the risk of type 2 diabetes mellitus. *Am J ClinNutr*. 2009;90:613-20.

44. Hu FB, Cho E, Rexrode KM, Albert CM, Manson JE. Fish and long-chain omega-3 fatty acid intake and risk of coronary heart disease and total mortality in diabetic women. *Circulation*. 2003;107:1852-7.

45. Willett W, MacMahon B. Diet and cancer—an overview. *N Engl J Med*. 1984;310:633-8.

46. Willett W, MacMahon B. Diet and cancer—an overview (second of two parts). *N Engl J Med*. 1984;310:697-703.

47. Smith-Warner S, Spiegelman D, Adami H, et al. Types of dietary fat and breast cancer: a pooled analysis of cohort studies. *Int J Cancer*. 2001;92:767-74.

48. Thiébaut A, Kipnis V, Chang S, et al. Dietary fat and postmenopausal invasive breast cancer in the National Institutes of Health-AARP Diet and Health Study cohort. *J Natl Cancer Inst*. 2007;99:451-62.

49. Cho E, Spiegelman D, Hunter D, et al. Premenopausal fat intake and risk of breast cancer. *J Natl Cancer Inst*. 2003;95:1079-85.

50. Sieri S, Krogh V, Pala V, et al. Dietary patterns and risk of breast cancer in the ORDET cohort. *Cancer Epidemiol Biomarkers Prev*. 2004;13:567-72.

51. Kushi L, Giovannucci E. Dietary fat and cancer. *Am J Med*. 2002;113Suppl 9B:63S-70S.

52. World Cancer Research Fund, American Institute for Cancer Research. Food, Nutrition, Physical Activity and the Prevention of Cancer: a Global Perspective – Online. 2007. Accessed January 11, 2012.

53. Zhang S, Hunter DJ, Rosner BA, Colditz GA, Fuchs CS, Speizer FE, Willett WC. Dietary fat and protein in relation to

risk of non-Hodgkin's lymphoma among women. *J Natl Cancer Inst*. 1999; 90:1751-8.

54. Lucas M, Mirzaei F, O'Reilly EJ, et al. Dietary intake of n-3 and n-6 fatty acids and the risk of clinical depression in women: a 10-y prospective follow-up study. *Am J ClinNutr*. 2011;93:1337-43.

55. Kruger MC, Coetzee M, Haag M, Weiler H. Long-chain polyunsaturated fatty acids: selected mechanisms of action on bone. *Prog Lipid Res*. 2010;49:438-49.

56. Parrott M, Greenwood C. Dietary influences on cognitive function with aging: from high-fat diets to healthful eating. *Ann N Y AcadSci*. 2007;1114:389-97.

57. Devore EE, Stampfer MJ, Breteler MM, et al. Dietary fat intake and cognitive decline in women with type 2 diabetes. *Diabetes Care*. 2009;32:635-40.

58. Hodge W, Schachter H, Barnes D, et al. Efficacy of omega-3 fatty acids in preventing age-related macular degeneration: a systematic review. *Ophthalmology*. 2006;113:1165-72.

59. Schwarz S, Leweling H. Multiple sclerosis and nutrition. *MultScler*. 2005;11:24-32.

60. Chavarro J, Rich-Edwards J, Rosner B, Willett W. Dietary fatty acid intakes and the risk of ovulatory infertility. *Am J Clin Nutr*. 2007;85:231-7.

61. Missmer SA, Chavarro JE, Malspeis S, et al. A prospective study of dietary fat consumption and endometriosis risk. *Hum Reprod*. 2010;25:1528-35.

62. Shai I, Schwarzfuchs D, Henkin Y, et al. Weight loss with a low-carbohydrate, Mediterranean, or low-fat diet. *N Engl J Med*. 2008;359:229-41.

63. Willett W, Stampfer M, Manson J, et al. Intake of trans fatty acids and risk of coronary heart disease among women. *Lancet*. 1993;341:581-5.

64. Vesper HW, Kuiper HC, Mirel LB, Johnson CL, Pirkle JL. Levels of plasma trans-fatty acids in non-Hispanic white adults in the United States in 2000 and 2009. *JAMA*.2012; 307:562-3.

65.www.ezinearticles.com

66.www.anykindapills.com